# Breast Enhancement Secrets and Myths from Around the World

## By Alexa Reyna

# COPYRIGHT © 2015 BY ALEXA REYNA

## DISCLAIMER

The content in this book is provided solely for informational purposes and is not to be viewed as a substitute for professional medical advice or to be relied upon for medication or treatment. Always seek the advice of your physician or other qualified health provider if you have questions regarding a medical condition. Never disregard medical advice or delay seeking it because of something you have read in this book. Neither the author nor anyone else associated with this book can be held accountable or liable, nor do they take any responsibly for any or all damage, injury, or consequence resulting from any attempt to use, misuse, adopt, or adapt any of the information presented in this book.

# ACKNOWLEDGEMENTS

I would like to thank all the women around the world who shared their culture's secrets and myths on natural breast enhancement. Ndikala in Cameroon, Kebrina in Jamaica, Yee in Malaysia, Ayesha in Pakistan, Ratna in Bangladesh, Katya in the Netherlands, Herminia in St Lucia, Nayana in Brazil, Claudia in Mexico, Shelah in Sweden, Oana in Romania, Jacqueline in Chile, Joy in Nigeria, and all the other wonderful women who made this book possible.

# PREFACE

I have always been interested in natural methods for breast enhancement and have been researching the topic for over a decade. In 2012, I decided to launch GrowBreastsNaturally.com to share with the world all that I've learned and continue to learn.

In recent years, my focus has been on Asian natural breast enhancement methods. There have been many success stories to come out of Asia and I wanted to know what they were doing to achieve such successes. I learned so many interesting things while researching Asian breast enhancement methods that I wondered what other myths, secrets, practices, and remedies were being performed or shared by women around the world. What I discovered was so remarkable that I felt it was necessary to compile and share this resource with all women.

*Breast Enhancement Secrets and Myths from Around the World* was written to introduce you to the world of natural breast enhancement and thus open your eyes to the various secrets, cultural beliefs, and myths of breast enhancement that have been passed down for generations.

I had the opportunity to speak to many wonderful women who shared with me their various cultural beliefs and practices. While reading this book, please keep in mind that these are the opinions or beliefs of only a sample of women from each country. They are the ideas and practices shared by mothers and daughters, passed down over time and may not necessarily represent the notions of the entire country from which these women and their beliefs originate.

My desire has always been to provide a concrete, web-based resource for natural breast enlargement via my website GrowBreastsNaturally. My hope is that this book will aid in the continuation of my mission by providing a worldwide perspective on natural breast enhancement. Throughout my many years of research, I have never come across such a unique compilation of breast enhancement information. I sincerely hope that you find the content in this book both entertaining and enlightening.

# TABLE OF CONTENTS

# INTRODUCTION

According to a 2012 United Nations statistical data report, there are approximately 3.48 billion females living in 229 countries throughout the world. While geographical location and cultural beliefs may set us apart, there is something we females all have in common: BREASTS, the universal sign of femininity.

Whether it is to feel more feminine, self-confident, or to attract a mate, the fact is a majority of women desire bigger breasts. For centuries, as far back as the Qing Dynasty in China when the Empress had a special pastry created in order to enhance her breasts to the ancient Ayurvedic methods that have been passed down for generations in India, a desire for larger breasts has existed.

In this book, you will discover breast enhancement secrets and myths from 30 countries. While many of the myths are derived from local plants and foods, as well as regional beliefs and customs, there are many secrets and myths that cross country borders, such as the use of massage or the consumption of soy products. Both are mentioned in a number of countries as a means for breast enhancement.

Not only will you learn methods to enhance your breasts, you will also discover each country's cultural beliefs around breasts and breast size.  By the time you finish reading this book, you will have a worldly view on breasts.  Now let's begin our journey.

# CHAPTER 1

❖

## ASIA

# BANGLADESH

Bangladeshi people think that enhanced breasts are a gift of the gods. Bangladeshi men prefer wives with big breasts at the time of their marriage. Some people believe that without sex, the breasts of a woman cannot be enhanced. Others believe that the more a woman has sex, the larger her breasts will become. There are also some people who have the opinion that if a woman drinks the water that comes from the sex organ of the male, her breasts are bound to be enhanced. Some people also say that if a man touches a woman's breasts, her breasts will grow.

**Breast Enlargement Folktale**

There is a known folktale on breast enhancement found in Bangladesh. It is as follows:

"There was once a village farmer that had a beautiful wife. She was perfect in every angle but she did not have large breasts. This made the husband sad. He would look at other men's wives and most days he would visit the brothels. As a result, his wife became very tense and went to a priest. The priest gave her "Ashwagandha" to enhance her breasts. She used it every morning and after a month, her breasts became so beautiful that the husband did not want to go to work and would rather spend the day with his wife."

This folktale inspired many women in Bangladesh to be more conscientious about beautifying their breasts.

## Foods for Breast Enhancement

Bangladesh is a country of vegetables and fruits. There are many different kinds of vegetables used by Bangladeshi women for the enlargement of the breasts. Some of these vegetables include: kidney beans, cauliflower, beets, broccoli, carrots, cucumber, tomatoes, mushrooms, Brussels sprouts, lentils, spring onions, celery, green beans, black eye peas, red beans, and chickpeas/garbanzo beans.

Consuming certain fruits are said to be beneficial to breast enhancement. Some of these fruits include: apples, plums, cherries, berries, pears, peaches, grapes, melons, raspberries, and blueberries.

Flaxseed is believed by many to be important in stimulating breast growth. Millet and barley are also helpful. Whole grains, brown rice, wheat germ, alfalfa sprouts, olives, prunes, and oats are also said to be good for breast enhancement.

## More Secrets and Myths

- Touching a man's penis on one's breasts will help enhance the breasts

- Applying cow dung on breasts is believed by some to help to increase the size of the breasts

- Punching and sucking breasts while having sex can enhance breast size

- Breastfeeding a child will increase breast size

# CHINA

The standard of beauty in old China included smaller breasts, but times have changed. The younger generations now desire to look more westernized with whiter skin, double eye-lids and bigger breasts.

China is home to 1.3 billion people and has one of the largest populations in the world. With so many people in one country, the pressure is huge to look beautiful and thus stand out. It is not all about vanity but about improving all aspects of their lives. Many Chinese are of the notion that looks are important for finding a job as well as a husband. As a result, cosmetic surgery is on the rise in China with procedures including nose jobs, double eye-lid surgery, chin jobs, and breast implants.

For those women who cannot afford surgery, ancient Chinese medicinal practices are utilized to increase breast size. Their natural breast enhancement regimens are truly an all-natural approach. They use their knowledge of the body and its energy systems, as well as the properties in food to trigger their breasts to grow.

**Acupressure**

Acupressure is based on the Traditional Chinese Medicine (TCM) practice of acupuncture. Acupressure is performed by applying pressure to acupoints, while acupuncture uses needles on these same points. Activating acupoints found throughout the body is said to balance the flow of energy to a specific area of the body and in turn, improve the health of that particular area. There are many acupoints that benefit the breasts which help to balance hormones and increase circulation as well as energy flow to the breasts.

**Breast Massage**

It is not uncommon in Asian cultures, particularly among the Chinese and Malaysian communities, for women to employ a professional masseuse to perform traditional breast massages which claim to enhance size, increase firmness, and tighten skin in the breast area.

This is common throughout China and a standard service offered at spas in the mainland. Modern spas in China often use a blend of time-tested traditional massage and modern technology.

Breast massage is said to alleviate the build-up of toxins as well as encourage healthy blood circulation and good lymphatic drainage. Sometimes breast masseurs are engaged by mothers who want to stimulate milk flow, an exercise which gained popularity after tainted milk scares in China.

**Breast Enhancing Pastry**

Legend has it that this pastry was created specifically for the Imperial Qing Dynasty Empress as a breast enhancer. The peanuts found in this pastry are high in protein and fat while the soy is high in phytoestrogens, or plant-based estrogen, and protein. Red dates are said to regulate the endocrine system and promote the development of breasts.

Ingredients:

100 grams peanuts

100 grams red dates, seeded

100 grams of soy

Instructions:

1. Preheat oven to 150 degree C (300 degrees F)
2. Remove skin from peanuts and soybeans and grind into powder
3. Add chopped dates to the mix, stir well
4. Add a little water and roll batter into balls
5. Press balls slightly to flatten out to desired thickness
6. Bake for 15 minutes.

**Breast Enhancing Tea**

According to legend, this tea is another item that was specifically developed for the Imperial Qing Dynasty Empress. Legend states that one should drink this tea while consuming the breast enhancing pastry above. Like the pastries, the jujubes, also known as red dates or Chinese dates, are believed to regulate the endocrine system and promote the development of breasts. Astragulus is believed to increase growth hormone levels as well as immunity and energy. This tea is also rumored to help reduce wrinkles.

Ingredients:

   3-5 pieces of Astragulus

   3 dates

   Water

Instructions:

1. Bring water to a boil

2. Add Astragulus pieces and dates

3. Seep and drink between meals

## Hasma

Another common urban legend among the Chinese is that consuming *Hasma* results in breast growth. *Hasma* is a delicacy made from the dried reproductive organs of a female frog, specifically the fatty tissue found near the fallopian tubes. This estrogen rich part of the frog is made into soups and stews as well as desserts in China. *Hasma* contains estrogen in large quantities – so much so that nutritionists recommend pre-pubescent children not consume *Hasma*.

# INDIA

India is a highly conservative society where any talk about breasts or breast size is frowned upon. But what cannot be denied is that breasts, like sex, are on everyone's mind in India and has been so for several centuries, despite protestations to the contrary.

Young, eligible men judge a prospective bride's suitability by slyly glancing at her well covered breasts and imagining. Mothers feed breast enhancement herbs recommended by the ancient Indian science of Ayurveda to their young pubescent daughters with the hope that their breasts will develop well, which in turn will help them get the right match when they are old enough for marriage.

While Indian society does not talk about it, for a young woman to have small breasts is akin to a curse in India. Some believe it indicates infertility and would make landing a suitable husband quite difficult. Often, young Indian women who have small breasts suffer from severe depression out of worry about the future.

Breast augmentation surgery hasn't really taken off in India as it has in western societies. This is why young women look to the ancient Indian medical science of Ayurveda for breast enlargement solutions. Ayurveda is recommended as an excellent natural breast enlargement solution, which does not require any invasive procedures to be made, has no serious side effects, and has been found to be highly effective by young Indian women over several centuries.

Below are a few popular Ayurveda herbs for breast enlargement, as well as the ideal diet recommended by Ayurveda for healthy growth of breasts and a couple of home remedies for breast enhancement, all based on the science of Ayurveda.

**Ayurvedic Herbs for Natural Breast Enhancement**

The following herbs have been recommended for centuries by Ayurvedic doctors in India for natural breast growth.

*Fenugreek* - Fenugreek is a very popular herb in India and has several benefits. One of these benefits is that fenugreek stimulates the breasts, helping with natural growth of the breasts.

*Lady's mantle* - Another popular natural breast growth herb is Lady's mantle. It is believed to increase blood flow to breast tissue and help maintain the breast fat deposits. It is recommended for well-proportioned breasts.

*Pueraria tuberosa* - Also known as kudzu, pueraria tuberosa is said to be a powerful, natural aphrodisiac. It is also said to work wonders for natural and healthy breast growth. It helps with larger and better proportioned breasts.

*Asparagus Racemosus* - Another popular Ayurvedic herb for breast enhancement is Asparagus racemosus, also known as shatavari. This herb is said to increase blood flow to the breasts and balance the hormonal system, all of which helps to enlarge the breasts naturally.

## Ayurvedic Diet for Natural Breast Enlargement

By incorporating certain changes to one's diet, it believed that one can experience a more wholesome breast growth.

Many women in India believe that having estrogen rich foods such as chicken head soup, dandelion root, watercress leaf, and carrots help with natural breast enlargement.

Drinking plenty of water and keeping constantly hydrated is important. Ayurveda considers water to be sacred and has several benefits, including being an excellent detoxifying agent, which helps in healthy breast enlargement.

Eating a lot of fruits and green vegetables is highly recommended. The fibrous content helps to detoxify the body and assists in healthy breast fat deposits in the breasts, resulting in more wholesome growth.

## Ayurveda Home Remedies for Natural Breast Growth

Several generations of Indian women have made use of the following Ayurvedic remedies, before passing them on to their young daughters.

## *Red Lentils (or Lens culinaris)*

Red lentils are believed to have remarkable breast enlargement powers. Women in India make a breast mask out of the red lentils to reap its breast enhancing benefits. They do this by soaking 15 grams of red lentils in lukewarm water for a couple of hours 'til they become soft. Then the women make a fine paste from them and apply the paste onto the breasts. The paste dries on the breasts for about 30 minutes. The paste is only to be applied and not massaged into the breasts. After 30 minutes, the dried paste is washed off thoroughly from the breasts. Indian Mothers have recommended this natural breast growth method to their young daughters for ages.

## *Natural Breast Growth Herbal Oil*

Another tradition for breast enhancement that has been passed down generations is massaging the breasts with essential oils. A popular homemade massage oil is made by adding 8 drops of Geranium essential oil and 15 drops of Ylang Ylang (Cananga odorata) to about 50 ml of almond oil. Women rub the oil mixture gently onto their breasts in a counter-clockwise massage, twice a day. It is believed that one will achieve great results in a couple of months or so, as long as it is done regularly.

# INDONESIA

Indonesia has one of the biggest Muslim populations in the world. The women there have the freedom to speak, work, dress, and drive just as men do, but when it comes to breasts as a topic of discussion, somehow it is still considered to be rather taboo. There are still quite a number of women who are shy when it comes to speaking about their own important body parts. Breasts are considered a private matter not to be exposed or spoken of. This does not mean that Indonesians do not value certain standards of breast beauty. This is apparent from the fact that there are numerous traditional beliefs, myths, secrets, and tips on how to enhance breasts naturally.

The following are several methods for natural breast enhancement found in Indonesia:

**Breast Masks and Massage Oils**

*Yard long bean* - Yard long beans are pureed and used as a breast mask. It is recommended that one apply the mix evenly on breasts (except the areola area) for about 30 minutes, at least 3 times a week. This method is said to be effective in enhancing and firming breasts.

*Fish oil* - is commonly used for massaging breasts.

*Shallot mix* - A mix of shallot, honey, and turmeric is said to be beneficial when applied on the breasts for about 30 minutes. This breast mask is said to enlarge breasts.

*Areca cathecu (Indonesian: Pinang)* - Areca cathecu is a palm tree that is native to Indonesia. Using the young fruit of this plant, also known as a Betel Nut or Areca Nut, is said to be effective for breast enhancement and a well-known myth in Indonesia. A mix of this palm fruit crushed with Daun Lempuyang (a local plant) and a pinch of salt is used as a mask for the breasts, except on the areola/nipples.

*Egg whites* - Egg white massage is believed to be beneficial to the breasts. The recipe states that one simply applies egg whites to the breasts and massages. The egg whites must be left on the breasts overnight to be effective. Rinse off in the morning.

*Cucumber* - This cucumber mask is said to enlarge breasts as well as soften the skin. Mash a cucumber and mix with lime and egg whites. Apply the mask on breasts and let sit for about 30 minutes then rinse off.

## Regular consumption of natural herbs/food/drink

*Sesbania grandiflora (Agati or Hummingbird Tree)* - Sesbania grandiflora, also known as *bunga turi* or *kembang turi* in Indonesian, is a small tree that is native to Southeast Asia. The leaves, flower, fruit, and bark of the tree are used as remedies for a variety of issues including headaches, fever, pain, and diarrhea. The flowers and leaves are also used in cooking.

There are two ways to use this plant to naturally enhance breasts. One way is to boil several of the flowers and drink as a tea. Another way is to cook the flowers as a main or side dish.

*Fresh milk and ginger mix* - One Indonesian myth for breast enhancement says to burn ginger and mix with fresh cow's milk. Let the mixture sit for 30 minutes to an hour then mix well and drink. The myth states that one should drink 1-2 times per day. Results should be expected in 2 – 4 weeks.

*Soybean* - Like many Asian countries, soybean consumption is believed by many in Indonesia to be an easy and delicious way to enhance breasts naturally. Soybeans can be consumed in a number of ways including tempeh, tofu, and soymilk.

# JAPAN

Since the early days of the kimonos, Japanese women have desired smaller breasts as a statement of beauty. Kimonos were designed to conceal the breasts and accentuate other parts of the body like the nape and waist. But as the years went on and Japan became more influenced by western culture, the desire for bigger, perfect breasts grew. Perfect breasts, as marketed to Japanese women, are those that are evenly round, face upwards and create a perfect equilateral triangle. This imaginary triangle is made between the nipples to the center of the collarbone. Bust measurements should also be equal or larger than the hips on an ideal body.

Achieving the perfect breasts is big business in Japan which has resulted in a number of breast enhancing services and products being marketed to women in Japan. Bust-up (*basuto appu*) is the Japanese term for breast enhancement which includes enlarging the breasts or changing their shape.

The Japanese expression *Bon Kyu Bon* translates as Good Small Good which equates to large bust, small waist, large hips, aka an hourglass figure. This concept is gaining more popularity than the thin/petite silhouette that was once desired in Japan.

## Esute Salons

Many *esute* or aesthetic salons in Japan offer bust-up treatments as a part of their menu of services. The treatment course for breasts generally consists of manual massage, application of creams, breast masks or mud packs, as well as stimulation provided by a mechanical device. These medical devices include vacuum or suction and/or electro-massage. The prices for these treatments are very expensive and for those who cannot afford these professional treatments, home remedies are utilized.

## Breast Care Salons

"Breast care salons" are salons or spas that focus only on the breasts. They provide breast enhancing treatments performed by the staff but also offer personal training and group seminars on bust-up products and techniques. Principles taught in these training sessions include: massage techniques, foods to eat and avoid, proper bra use, as well as exercises and other tips that one can implement at home to naturally increase breast size.

## Massage and Fat Brushing

Massage is a very important part of the Japanese bust-up system. Specific massage techniques are used to drain the lymphatic system as well as increase circulation to the breasts. Fat brushing is a popular massage technique used to migrate fat from one part of the body to the breasts. Over time, with proper use of a bra, the fat is believed to stay in the breasts, giving them a fuller, perkier shape.

**Shiatsu**

*Shiatsu* is the Japanese variation of Chinese acupuncture. It uses many of the same techniques and pressure points used in Chinese acupuncture. By activating certain *shiatsu* points on the body, the following benefits are said to be gained:

- relieve pain in the breasts
- increase milk supply
- increase circulation and energy in the breasts

**Breast Enhancement Legend - Chiyomilk**

Chiyomilk is a legendary female who had much success with the Japanese bust-up method. She reportedly went from a C to H/I cup (B to F/G cup in US sizes) in a span of 3 years. Her routine consisted of taking breast enhancing supplements like pueraria mirifica and pig placenta. She also massaged her breasts and used the fat brushing technique to move fat from her stomach and back to her breasts. Her journey has been well documented on her blog and includes many before and after pictures.

**Breast Shrines and Temples**

Ōkunitama Jinja Shinto shrine is located in Fuchu City, Japan. Many mothers visit the shrine to pray for good breast milk but it has recently become known as the "Bust-Up Shrine". This is due to an ancient gingko tree that is located behind the shrine. Many women go there to pray for bigger breasts while some believe that if you touch the tree, and then touch your breasts with the same hand, it will give your breasts a boost.

*Mamachichi Kannon* or *Mama Kannon* (formally known as *Ryuuon-ji*) located in Aichi Prefecture is a Buddhist temple known as the "Breast Temple." This temple is dedicated to *Kannon*, the Buddha of Mercy, and was founded in 1492. The temple grounds are full of breast sculptures and one can purchase *Emas* (wooden wishing plaques) to write their wishes for bigger breasts and leave at the temple.

# MALAYSIA

Malaysia is a multiracial country. It has a population of 23.27 million consisting of 60 percent Malays, 30 percent Chinese, 8 percent Indians, and 2 percent other ethnic groups. Malaysia is unique because of its diversity of races, religions, and cultures, the stability of the country and many places of interests. Below are some secrets and myths from each racial group found in Malaysia.

**Malay:**

One myth involves using "daun sirih melayu" (aka Betel) and putting a few drops of coconut oil on top of leaves. Heat it up with a candle and when the oil is warm enough, put the mix on the breasts and leave it on the breasts until the oil is absorbed by the skin. Repeat this a few times a week.

Another myth says to spread egg whites onto the breasts and leave on until the next morning. Repeat the process at least one more time within two days.

A popular breast exercise to increase breast size is to first, stand up straight. Then, place both hands on opposite breasts and press breasts against each other and release. Continue the exercise for 10 – 15 minutes.

This pumpkin breast mask is said to be beneficial to breast enhancement. Simply peel and cook a whole pumpkin until its tender. While it's still warm, mash the pumpkin and spread it onto the breast. Leave the mask on the breasts for 20 minutes and rinse. Twice a week is recommended for this myth.

**Chinese:**

Drink a lot of soymilk.

Eat chicken to enlarge your breast.

Eat a lot of papaya or drink papaya milkshakes, which are very common in the Chinese community.

Let your breasts be as free as possible at all times either by wearing a loose bra or no bra at all. This is said to help facilitate breast growth since the breasts are not constrained and the tissue is allowed to expand more easily on its own without any restrictions.

Massage your breast 3 times a day. It is said to increase blood and lymph flow to the region. Sesame oil is recommended by many for breast massage.

In traditional Chinese medicine, star anise is prescribed as a digestive aid. It is also believed to promote health of female reproductive organs and is recommended for lactating mothers to increase breast milk secretion. As a result, many believe it is also beneficial for increasing breast size.

Chinese herbal remedies such as dong quai and bird's nest are said to have breast enhancing effects.

## Indian:

Daily massage with fennel seeds and oil is said to increase breast size. Fennel seeds contain a high content of flavonoids which are believed to increase estrogen levels in the body.

Many Indian women believe that spices like fenugreek powder can promote estrogen levels. One way women use fenugreek powder is to soak the powder overnight in a cup of water and drink the mixture in the morning.

Sesame seed and flaxseed are said to be beneficial to breast enhancement. These are easily added to one's diet by sprinkling onto their meal.

Indian women believe that eating a lot of papaya during puberty helps to enhance breast growth but it is also believed that the breasts will become papaya-shaped.

# PAKISTAN

In some parts of Pakistan, heavier women are considered attractive because it is considered a sign of healthy living. A more common belief is that breasts are considered a symbol of beauty and add to the figure of a woman. Mothers in Pakistan generally educate their daughters about breasts, especially in their growing age. A common myth that is passed down to young girls is that sour things are the real breast enhancers, if they are used properly at the ideal age.

## Breast Enhancement in Pakistan

The rate of girls who want larger breasts in Pakistan is increasing day by day. The following are a couple of reasons why some women attempt natural breast enhancement.

- Some women in Pakistan want larger breasts because their husbands, boyfriends, or fiancés demand it.

- Others desire an increase in their breast size because they want to embrace their femininity and show that their figure is a well-shaped figure.

Some natural remedies used by Pakistani women to achieve enhanced breasts are:

**Sour foods**

An important method used by girls in Pakistan for increasing the breast size is eating sour things like Tamarind (*imli*). If a girl takes the proper amount of tamarind or other sour food during the ages of 13 through 15, it is said that she will surely get the best results. This method is said to not be as effective in older aged women. It is a common myth that has been passed down through generations in Pakistan.

**Massage**

Like many countries, massaging the breasts is a very common method for breast enhancement. Among Pakistani women, it is believed to be an easy and effective way to increase breast size. During this process, girls apply a lotion or cream and massage the breasts in a circular motion. The belief is that the breast massage will produce heat and breast cells will propagate. The massage on the right breast should be done clockwise while the motion should be counter-clockwise on the left breast.

**Tight bra**

There is another myth is Pakistan which states that breast size can be increased by wearing a tight bra. In order for it to work, the bra should be tight around the bottom, while the cups of the bra should be large enough to give space for the breasts to grow.

## Warmth

Sometimes ladies in Pakistan use warm clothes or warm water to increase the temperature of the blood in the breast which is believed to increase the size of the breasts.

# PHILLIPINES

In the 10th century, the Ifugao people in the northern Philippines especially cared about the size of a woman's breasts when she was about to be married. The size of the breasts determined the size of the dowry to be given to the man's family.

Today, in many areas of the Philippines, especially those dominated by Islamic influence, large breasts are considered undesirable. As a result, selling breast enhancers or providing natural treatments for breast enlargement are frowned upon.

In the larger cities, western influence has helped women see their breasts as an aspect of femininity which has resulted in the desire for bigger breasts for a small few.

Some of the few natural treatments used by Filipinas to enhance the size of their breasts include eating papaya, avocadoes, and jicama (known locally as *singkamas*). These foods are said to contain nutrients that enhance the production of fatty tissue on the breasts. They also prevent darkening of the areola due to their natural whitening properties.

# SOUTH KOREA

Until recent years, South Korean societal views on larger breasts have carried negative connotations such as associating women with larger breasts with being intellectually inferior or being promiscuous, hence not a desirable attribute when seeking a mate. It was actually considered embarrassing if one had big breasts. However, more interest in larger breasts now exists due to recent western influences. This is especially true in ad media post the 1990's when the ban on western lingerie models was lifted and they were allowed to use full body poses compared to Korean lingerie models that were photographed from the neck down due to the shame factor.

A thin figure with big breasts now is representative of beauty in present day South Korea. It is common to find television shows demonstrating to women how they can shape their body and enhance their breasts naturally. Breast implant surgeries are on the rise in Korea but so is the use of natural methods to fulfill the desire of bigger breasts. Below are common beliefs regarding natural breast enhancement in South Korea.

**Hip Baths**

It is recommended that women keep their female organs warm. This includes the ovaries and breasts. It is believed that if your organs are cold, hormone balance is broken and blood circulation is bad. As a result, nutrients and hormones from the ovaries do not reach the breasts. You can simply warm up your ovaries and breasts by taking a bath. If that is not an option, another way Korean women maintain warmth to the ovaries is to take "hip baths". Hip baths are similar to regular baths but on a much smaller scale. You will need a big bucket or container, one that your bottom can fit in. Fill it with warm water and sit just your bottom in it. Some women put herbs in the water to enhance the benefits of the bath.

**Strawberry Milk**

A common myth for those desiring bigger breasts is that drinking strawberry milk will help. The strawberry milk myth for enlarging breasts was popularized by a cable television show called Martian X File, which on December 28th 2012, featured two sisters who drank 30 packs of strawberry milk (250ml each) everyday while also using milk to bathe in and eating ramen with milk. The sisters claim to have gone from a size A cup to an E as a result. The belief is that the strawberries' breast enlarging effects come from its plant-based estrogen content while the milk is high in nutritional value.

**Carrots**

Carrots are believed to help prevent breast sagging as well as help beautify the breast shape. It is recommended that one eats raw carrots to receive these effects. Carrots that have been cooked are said to have lost their breast beautifying qualities.

## Pomegranate

This super food is full of antioxidants which is great for the skin and is said to help reduce the risk of cancer. But in South Korea, many believe that this super fruit is beneficial to the breasts because of its phytoestrogen rich content.

## Collagen

Eating collagen rich foods is said to be beneficial to the elasticity of the breast tissue. Collagen is believed to strengthen the connective tissue of the breasts which helps to reduce sagging. Some of the collagen rich foods eaten in South Korea are: pig feet, pig skin, chicken feet, sea cucumber, and sea squirt (mong-gae). Collagen powders and tablets are also available and popular in South Korea.

## Soymilk

Like many Asian countries, the consumption of soymilk and other soy products are popular among Korean women for breast growth. Soy contains high levels of plant-based estrogens, specifically isoflavones, which are believed to help breast grow.

## Breast Enhancing Herbs

A number of herbs are used by women in Korea to balance hormones as well as increase blood circulation and improve the health of the uterus, all of which are believed to be beneficial to breast enhancement. Some of these herbs include:

- Angelica Root (Dong Quai)
- Burdock Root
- Cnidium
- Evening Primrose Oil
- Fenugreek
- Flaxseeds
- Pueraria Lobata (Kudzu)
- Pueraria Mirifica
- Saw palmetto
- Wild Yam

## North Korean breast beliefs

Large breasts are negatively viewed in North Korea, similar to how it was in South Korea not too long ago. According to a North Korean expat blogger, women in North Korea who have large breasts are viewed as flirts and having bigger breasts is something women should be ashamed of. As a result, well-endowed women in North Korea generally try to hide their breasts and some even try natural means to make their breasts smaller. One rumored fix is the consumption of chives.

# TAIWAN

Like many Asian countries, thin and petite was once considered beautiful in Taiwan. And like many Asian countries, the standards of beauty have evolved to reflect western ideals. Taiwan's new standard of beauty includes white skin, large breasts, and colored eyes as well as tall and thin yet curvy bodies. Taiwan is only 100 miles off the coast of China. Their relative proximity and intertwined histories have resulted in much Chinese influence, particularly in regard to the breast enhancement practices and beliefs of Taiwanese women. Many of the techniques used in Taiwan are based on Traditional Chinese Medicine (TCM) principles.

**Chinese Food Therapy / Dietary Therapy**

Chinese food therapy, also known as dietary therapy or nutritional therapy, is a TCM practice that uses food to heal or maintain good health. The basic idea around Chinese food therapy is that each food has a *Yin* or *Yang* property also known as hot or cold. This is not hot or cold as in temperature but as in the type of energy the food carries. In order to heal the body, or in this case grow breasts naturally, one must eat more foods of one property and less of those with the other.

## Green Papaya

A popular idea in Taiwanese society is that papayas – especially green ones – are the key to growing an ample bosom. There are many recipes for green papayas and many mothers encourage their daughters to eat green papayas. It is believed to be more effective at breast growth for young women compared to older women. Green papaya is also eaten by new mothers as it assists them with the production of milk.

An old wives' tale states that brewing green papaya and pork ribs soup was the key to helping young women grow larger breasts. A more modern take is the papaya milkshake made with ripe, sweet papayas. It is sold in night markets across the country. The humble papaya milkshake is credited with helping young girls achieve a flawless complexion and yes, the highly coveted bigger breasts.

### Green Papaya and Pork Ribs Soup

Ingredients:

1 small-to-medium green papaya

500g diced pork ribs

2 small pieces of fresh ginger

1 carrot and sliced cabbage for garnish

Water

Instructions:

1. Clean the pork ribs

2. Put the ribs and ginger in a pot with 2 liters of water.

3. Bring to a boil then reduce the heat. Let it simmer for 90 minutes.

4. Peel the skin on the green papaya and remove the seeds. Cut into cubes.

5. Dice or slice carrots as per your preference.

6. Put carrot and papaya cubes into the pot.

7. Season with salt and white pepper powder to taste. Once the papaya is soft, you can serve.

## Chicken Feet

Chicken feet are a favored snack prepared by street vendors throughout Taiwan. It is also another popular food item for those wanting to attain larger breasts. Chicken feet are rich in protein, calcium, and collagen. The breasts are made of connective tissue which provides support and helps give breasts their shape. The collagen in chicken feet is said to help strengthen the connective tissue in the breasts. Chicken feet are also eaten by many for their cosmetic benefits. The collagen present in chicken feet is said to increase skin elasticity and reduce winkles. Eating chicken feet is also believed to minimize arthritis and joint pain. Chicken feet are prepared fried or sautéed and eaten in soups and broths as well.

# THAILAND

Thailand is a country rich in herbal products. Since ancient times, Thai people have been using herbs to cure diseases and treat imperfections of the body. The Thais have also grown up with some beliefs and taboos. Some women still trust natural methods for treating their beauty, including enlarging their breasts.

## Pueraria Mirifica

Pueraria mirifica (aka the Miracle Herb) is an herbal plant that only grows in Thailand, mainly the northern area. Women in Thailand have been using this plant for generations for its anti-aging and rejuvenating power. In recent years, it has become very popular throughout the world for its natural breast enhancing properties. Pueraria mirifica contains the highest levels of phytoestrogens which is said to help breasts grow. It is such a hit in Japan that they have created breast enhancement cookies and gum made of pueraria mirifica.

## Thai Breast Slapping

Breast slapping is a method of delivering rhythmic, kneading slaps to a woman's breast to increase the size and improve firmness. A study by the Thai Health Ministry found that the vigorous massage left volunteers' breasts measurably bigger. The Ministry even sponsored a program that supported women learning to slap their own breasts to enhance their size as an alternative to surgery.

This technique claimed to visibly increase the cup size of clients after just one session. There is no surgery involved at all, just a lot of kneading and pummeling. Therapists claim that the technique works by shifting fat from one area to another, and vigorously kneading excess fat towards the breast area. Some therapists who specialize in this treatment have expanded their practice to include "buttock-slapping" to increase butt size and "face slapping" to help reduce wrinkles and tighten skin.

### Chicken Breast

Some women in Thailand believe that eating a lot of chicken breasts from hens will powerfully enhance breasts of young girls during their reproductive age. Some believe this method can be harmful as the chickens have been given growth hormones to hasten their growth and size and should not be eaten by humans.

### Breast Massage

A common belief in Thailand is that constant massaging of the breasts with herbal oil will stimulate breast growth. Massaging is said to increase the flow of blood to the breasts which results in increased firmness.

## Birth Control Pills

Most Thai teenagers (female and "ladyboy") believe that taking birth control pills can boost their breast size. Many use the pill without consulting a doctor, which can be harmful.

# VIETNAM

The topic of breasts in Vietnam, like many other Asian countries, is a very sensitive topic. As a result, Vietnamese do not have many secrets or myths about breast or breast enhancement but they do have a few. The Vietnamese believe that food is the key to growing breasts without pills. Here are some foods that they believe help breasts grow:

## Green Papaya and Pig Feet Soup:

Green papaya and pig feet soup is a traditional recipe used by Vietnamese women to enhance breasts. Pig feet contain protein and are rich in collagen while green papaya is a well-known secret for breast enhancement.

## Peanut with Chicken Feet and Ginger Soup

Peanut with chicken feet and ginger soup is believed to help increase breast size. The peanuts are said to be a rich source of estrogen and protein while chicken feet, like pigs feet, contain protein and collagen, all of which are said to be beneficial to breast growth.

## BBQ Pig or Goat Breast

Vietnamese believe that the organs you eat from animals will be beneficial to your organs. For example, if you eat a pig heart, it will be good for your heart. So if you eat a pig or goat breast, it will be good for your breasts. This is similar to glandular therapy which is a popular form of breast enhancement in the United States where women consume animal glandulars, such as bovine ovary pills, to increase breast size.

## Soya Milk

A common belief among Vietnamese women is that drinking plenty of soya milk is beneficial to breast enhancement. It is believed to boost hormone levels because of the estrogen found in soya or soy.

## Boiled Peanuts

Vietnamese women believe that while you are on your menstrual cycle, your breasts are generally very tender and bigger than normal. A Vietnamese myth states that if you eat a lot of boiled peanut during this time, your breasts will stay this size all the time.

## Unpadded Bras

Many Vietnamese women believe that teenagers who are going through puberty should not wear thick padded bras because they will restrict their breasts and cause them to stop growing. The padded bras are believed to even make their breasts smaller.

# CHAPTER 2

❖

# EUROPE

# BULGARIA

The top three things most Bulgarians take pride in, would almost certainly be: their history, their yogurt, and their beautiful women. According to statistical data, as a mix of different genotypes, the modern Bulgarian woman is typically 5.5 feet tall and relatively slim with an average bust size of 32" (bra cup D). Is there a special secret to achieving such impressive breast size? You can seek an answer in the many recipes, procedures, ancient wisdoms, and pure fantasies shared among Bulgarian women.

## Breast Enhancing Foods

There are a number of foods, herbs, and spices which are believed to benefit healthy and natural breast growth:

*Flaxseed* - Consumed ground or in the form of oil, flaxseed is said to be beneficial for female hormonal balance and thus, for breast growth.

*Dill* - A traditional part of Bulgarian cuisine is also believed to assist in obtaining a bigger chest size naturally.

*Fenugreek* - A common herb widely used in Bulgaria, fenugreek seed sprouts can be added to salads or consumed as tea.

*Barm* - Besides maintaining the health of a women's skin and nails, barm is believed by some to be beneficial for growing bigger breasts.

*Hop vine* - Some swear by this grain's ability to provide one with rounder and larger breasts within about 12 weeks of consistent consumption.

## Beinsa Douno Method

Peter Deunov (also known as Beinsa Douno), a renowned Bulgarian healer and spiritual leader, suggests the following "cure" for flat chested ladies:

Syrup prepared from:

2 oz plantain leaves

3 tbps parsley roots

2 tbps ground fenugreek seed

1 lemon (squeezed and its peels rasped)

1 tbps cocoa

18 oz honey

Bring mixture to a boil and simmer for 30 minutes, filter, and keep in the fridge. One spoonful is to be taken 3 times per day, 20 minutes prior to eating.

10 minutes after eating the above syrup, one consumes a glass of the following concoction:

36 oz water from boiled walnuts

2 tbps each - Eryngium campestre (sea holly), Restharrow root and nettle

1 tbps each - chicory roots, barley and oat grains

The mixture is boiled for 15 minutes in 101 oz water. 4 tablespoons of the following blend is added to the mixture:

2oz each of:

Pine tips

White mulberry leaves

Iceland moss

Fumaria officinalis

Flores Helichrysi

Spiraea ulmaria (Meadowsweet)

Hop vine

After 15 more minutes of boiling, the syrup is filtered and taken with honey and lemon for better taste.

For breast enhancement, Daunov also suggests putting fresh cabbage leaves on the breasts overnight.

## More Secrets and Myths

*Cold Water* - is said to be a female bosom's best friend. Breasts look enhanced when the skin is kept young and firm. Contrast showers (switching between hot and cold water) is one way to achieve this. Another option is to rub ice on your décolleté after a shower.

*Massage* - Massaging breasts with a soft brush for 5 minutes each morning is also believed to be a way to achieve an enhanced bust. The massage is said to stimulate muscle and tissue growth, enlarging the breasts and helping them stay perky.

*Posture* - Standing and sitting with a straight back and raised shoulders makes the breasts look bigger. Chest stretching exercises are also said to help.

## Superstitions

Some Bulgarian women believe that if a pregnant woman's breasts grow faster than her belly, she is having a girl. If the belly grows faster than the breasts, she is having a boy.

It may sound cruel but some believe that if a baby girl is left to cry longer, she will have bigger breasts when she grows up.

Another Bulgarian superstition involves breasts and dreams. If one has a dream involving beautiful woman's breasts, he may expect a pleasant surprise in the future. However, if the breasts are small, poverty or grief is coming.

Many Bulgarian women desire larger breasts because they believe larger sized breasts will make them look more attractive and feel more confident. Many women post-pregnancy are less concerned about achieving larger sized breasts and more interested in firmer, better looking ones.

For the above reasons, breast enhancement surgery is still one of the most common plastic surgeries performed in the country. But there are still women who do not dare have it done out of fear that the potential breast cancer would be harder to detect or that they will be unable to breastfeed a child later in life.

# FRANCE

In general, France is fond of smaller breasts compared to the United States or Italy. When interviewed, a former Miss France said, "Small breasts aregood because we can always cheat about the size. You can always make them look bigger whenever you want (and not the opposite), and I like it!"

Since breast enlargement is not big in France, many of the secrets and myths are basic know how.

## Chest Exercises

The development of the pectoral muscles under the breast can be made through regular muscle strengthening exercises. This can help improve the size and the firmness of the breast.

## Gain Weight

If one is thin, French women believe one should consider gaining weight. The breast is composed mainly of fatty connective tissue. Like the rest of adipose tissue in the body, it may be lost when a woman loses weight. If you are thin and have small breasts, gaining a few kilos of fat is suggested to help fill out your chest.

## Stand up Straight

French women believe something simple as standing up straight can give your breasts a visual boost. Some women find that their breasts appear smaller than they really are when they do not stand in a straight position. To enhance your breasts immediately, just stand up straight! Stand up straight, keep your head up and put your shoulders back. Keep your neck vertical - do not let it fall forward.

## Birth Control Pills

Breast augmentation is a known side effect of many hormone-based oral contraceptives. This can be explained by the fact that most birth control pills affect hormones levels which may result in a slight increase of the breasts. Thus, it is believed by many that taking birth control pills will result in bigger breasts. For women who want to avoid an unwanted pregnancy and coincidentally also wish to have bigger breasts, birth control pills are believed by some to be an effective solution.

# GREECE

Breast enhancement is not a common practice among everyday women in Greece. It is more likely to be seen among celebrities and public figures. In ancient Greece, it was not a vulgar or uncommon thing to see a woman's breast on display per se, such as it is today. Greeks today have become more conservative when it comes to a female's breasts than the times of the Minoan civilization. The following are a few home remedies a Greek grandmother might recommend:

- Use yogurt and oat bran to make a mask for firming your breasts

- For firmer breasts, use chamomile oil with a touch of lavender oil and massage for about 3 minutes

- For bigger breasts, drink a cup of sage

- Eating lot of chicken breast (protein) will aid in breast enlargement

# ITALY

The breasts are certainly the part of the female physique that first enchants an Italian man. Throughout the history of this country, breasts have been called by different pet names, some of which are "poppe," "zizze," and others a bit more vulgar.

Every man in Italy dreams of falling asleep on a breast and women are well aware of this. For this reason, many Italian women tend to treat their breasts and enhance their shape through the use of various stratagems to make them even more beautiful without losing their naturalness. It is said that in ancient times the Italian women used treatments based on alchemilla (lady's mantle), fenugreek, galega (goat's rue), or serpollino (wild thyme) to keep the breast elastic and firm.

In addition, the herbalist tradition followed by Italian women over centuries report many applications for natural breast care. The most popular ones known by Italian women of the past, so-called "grandma's remedies," are as follows:

- Massage with almond oil supplemented with mint extract and sage

- Make a cold compress with an infusion of serpollino, thyme, and rosemary cooled for 15 minutes

- Breast mask composed of olive oil and egg yolk

- Increase breast size by drinking milk and eating dairy products

- Flaxseed is an ideal remedy to tone and increase breast size

- Pepper, thyme, and fennel eaten as a compress / infusion is said to be ideal for improving the appearance of the breast

# NETHERLANDS

According to Anatole France, "A woman without breasts is like a bed without pillows." But that's just the 20th century opinion of a French man. His 21st century European Dutchman, however, prefer a different saying: "Quality over quantity."

Most Dutch women value their health and comfort above all. They are active and confident. It is not that beauty is not important to them but what is valued there is a more natural and casual look. One may call it "bicycle magnificence" because most Dutch use their bikes to get around and as a result are largely fit, tall, and good-looking.

According to Target Map, the average woman's bra cup size is D. Is it the Dutch cheese, the active lifestyle, or a combination of factors that helped achieve such breast size? Here are a few Dutch secrets for enhanced breasts which may give a clue:

**Breast Masks**

For a beautiful and firm décolleté, Dutch women count mostly on natural masks, teas, and smoothies. Best of all, most ingredients are easily found in every kitchen.

*Fermented Milk Breast Mask*

3 drops of ylang ylang essential oil

3.5 oz probiotic fermented milk (Yakult)

Massage mask onto the breasts for 2 minutes. Leave breast mask on for additional 5 minutes then rinse with warm water.

*Watermelon and green papaya mask*

This mask is believed to enhance blood flow and make the skin firm and radiant.

1 tbsp flour

1 small serving of green papaya

1 small serving of watermelon

2 drops of geranium essential oil

Put the fruits in a blender then mix the blended fruit with the oil and the flour. Massage the breasts with the mixture for 2 minutes and leave on breasts for 15 additional minutes. Rinse with warm water.

The longer the skin is massaged when applying the above mask, the more effectively the ingredients are said to be absorbed by the skin. The masks activate cell renewal and improve blood flow, thus aiding in natural breast growth.

**Fenugreek**

Fenugreek is not only good for breast enhancement but it also aids in digestion and immune system health. 1-2 cups per day of fenugreek tea is believed to bring good results when it comes to breast enhancement.

To make the tea, boil one cup of fenugreek seeds or sprouts and a handful of fennel seed, also beneficial for breast growth, in two cups of water.

A fenugreek herbal capsule can also be mixed with olive or grape seed oil and used as a mask on the breasts. This method is even better for boosting healthy breast growth because all nutrients are absorbed directly through the skin instead of being processed by the liver.

**Smoothies with Soymilk**

Smoothies are a refreshing way to achieve better looking breasts and skin, as well as boost energy. Combining vitamin rich fruits of your choice with soymilk is yet another thing Dutch women do for achieving beautiful breasts. Soy is a good source of plant-based proteins and phytoestrogens which help with breast growth.

**More Secrets and Myths**

Besides regular massages with natural ingredients and essential oils, Dutch women do their best to maintain a healthy weight. In addition to biking, they exercise a few times per week to prevent a sagging bosom and promote steady estrogen levels.

The Dutch diet is rich in milk products – cheeses, yogurt, and desserts. Peanuts, consumed in the form of butter or sauce, are known to aid the impressive Dutch height, health, and beauty.

One thing that is not widely spread amongst the Dutch is irrational or negative thinking. Perhaps hearty living and optimism are the two things most needed not only for happiness but also for beautiful breasts?

# POLAND

The Polish society is quite conservative. This viewpoint is largely found in smaller cities and villages. The perspective in the big cities is quite different with a more open point of view when it comes to breasts. For example, there is an increase of breast enhancement operations in the bigger cities compared to the smaller. But in general, Polish women desire to be slim and have good body proportions. Overall, Polish women respect themselves and their bodies, and are generally healthy.

## B Vitamins

The consumption of foods which contain vitamin B, such as buckwheat and walnuts, are believed to help increase breast size. Vitamin $B_5$ is responsible for the production of sex hormones, while $B_3$ is involved in the synthesis of sex hormones and $B_{12}$ is said to increase libido and fertility.

## Exercise

Swimming regularly for 10 minutes a day to strengthen chest muscles is recommended to reduce sagging in the breasts. Stretching exercises for the upper part of the body are said to also be beneficial to the breasts.

## Cold Water

Some women claim that washing your breasts with cold water in the mornings and evenings will help reduce sagging and make the breasts look fuller. The water must be as cold as you can withstand. For those who are brave enough, rubbing your breasts with snow is said to produce the same benefit.

## Breast Massage

Massaging your breasts with honey is said to give excellent results. Honey is also known to restore the skin collagen and delay the effects of aging.

Another massage that is said to be beneficial to the breasts is to rub the breasts with warm water, vinegar, and salt in the evenings. Afterwards, rinse the breasts with cool water and start massaging gently with olive or lemon juice. Massage the breasts in a circular motion, inward from the body to the center of the chest. This massage can be performed lying down or while in the shower.

## Breast Enhancing Tea

The following mix is said to help enhance breasts. Mix fenugreek, dill, anise, licorice, and cumin with water and boil. Drink this mix 1-2 times a day. Results are said to show in a few weeks.

## More Secrets and Myths

Eating a lot of bananas and chocolate is said to aid in breast enlargement. Contact with semen on one's breasts is also rumored to help them grow.

# PORTUGAL

Portugal is a laid back country with very open-minded people especially when it comes to sex and appreciating their women. Portuguese women are very feminine and take good care of themselves. They are also generally curvy. Portuguese men like their women this way, with nice breasts, buttocks, and a small waist.

**Ways to Firm Your Breasts:**

- Take cold water showers or massage the breasts with ice

- Beat an egg white until stiff. Put the mixture on your breasts and let sit for 30 minutes. Rinse off with water.

- Chest exercises like pushups are said to strengthen chest muscles which reduce sagging in the breasts.

**Breast Masks**

*Yogurt and egg mask*

Ingredients:

1 plain yogurt

1 egg

1 tspn of vitamin E oil

Instructions:

1. Mix all the ingredients together.

2. Rub the mixture on the breasts. Massage with circular movements for about 3 minutes then put an old bra on over the breasts.

3. Let sit for about 25 minutes. Wash off with warm water.

*Apple Mask*

This is a traditional recipe with confirmed results, so they say.

Ingredients:

2 apples

750 ml milk

Instructions:

1. Cut the apples and remove seeds. Chop apples well.

2. Put milk into a pot and bring to a boil.

3. Add the pieces of apple and cook until it is a thick mass.

4. Let mix cool then apply onto the breasts.

5. Remove after 15 minutes. Wash with warm water then with cold water.

*Banana Mask*

This mask is rumored to prevent sagging and make your breasts look like they did when you were a teen. It can be made every day until you see results.

Ingredients:

Fully ripe bananas

Instructions:

1. Mash the quantity of bananas that you think will be sufficient to cover both breasts entirely.

2. Massage mashed bananas on to breasts in a circular motion.

3. Let it stand for at least 30 minutes. Wash off with cold water.

*Cucumber Mask*

This mask is said to strengthen tissue around the breast area.

Ingredients:

1 cucumber

1 egg yolk

Butter cream

Instructions:

1. Mash the cucumber.

2. Add egg yolk and a little butter cream.

3. Mix well and apply on the breast.

4. Leave for on for 15-20 minutes. Rinse off with cold water.

*Lemon Egg Yolk Mask*

This mask is said to improve and protect breast skin.

Ingredients:

½ lemon

1 egg yolk

Instructions:

1. Mix juice from half a lemon and the lemon peel (without the white part of the peel) with an egg yolk. Consistency should be a paste.

2. Apply paste to breasts in circular movements, avoiding the nipples.

3. Leave on for 15-20 minutes then wash paste off with cold water.

## Breast Massage

Massaging with the following concoctions are said to help firm the skin around the breasts and to give a smooth look to the breasts:

*Lemon & Rum*

Mix 1 lemon and 1/2 cup of good quality rum. Let mixture stand overnight. The next day, massage breasts with the lemon rum mix.

*Parsley & Butter*

Let stand for 30 minutes then wash off.

## Massage with Oils

It is recommended that one should massage the breasts at least 2-3 times a week using olive oil. This will help the skin stay firm and improve the tone and texture. It will also improve skin elasticity.

Massage with different oils for different skin types at least 3 times per week. The oils include the following:

*Borage oil* - Borage works especially well on dry skin to preserve collagen fibers which provide elasticity.

*Wheat germ oil* - Especially for dehydrated and/or damaged breasts. It is soothing, nourishing, and anti-wrinkle.

*Evening primrose oil* - For delicate skin. Ensures the regeneration of collagen fibers and prevents the appearance of wrinkles.

*Avocado oil* - For cracked, dehydrated, and weak skin. Protects the skin and increases elasticity.

Additional oils used by Portuguese women for breast massage are almond oil and grape seed oil.

## Ice Massage

Ice massage is believed by many Portuguese women to be a very effective way to eliminate sagging of the breasts. With two ice cubes, one for each breast, make circular motions around your chest for at least a minute. Not more than that is recommended as the skin on the breast is very sensitive.

An alternative to the ice massage is to use cold water. It is believed to be very effective in maintaining healthy and cheerful breasts if you apply every day. Similar to the ice method, massage breasts with cold water in circular movements. This can be done simply by massaging your breasts while taking a cold shower.

## Exercise

Similar to the beliefs of women in France and Poland, one of the best ways to firm the breasts is by doing chest exercises. The best choice is push-ups, which help the pectoral muscles under the breast. It is also said to shape the breasts and reduce sagging around the chest.

## Foods to Eat

Below are a list of foods Portuguese women believe have breast enhancing properties.

*Flaxseed* - One should eat a good portion of flaxseed (30 to 50 grams) every day. Flaxseed can be added to salads or some just mashed into a cup of water or milk.

*Soy* - is a beneficial food for breast enlargement. One can add soy to meals or drink a cup of soymilk. Tofu is also another good source of soy.

*High fiber foods* - High fiber foods like oats, wheat, or barley can also help to enlarge breasts.

*Fenugreek and wild yam* – are said to contribute to natural breast enlargement and are said to also be used as sexual stimulants.

*Sesame seeds* - It is said to be a must-have in one's diet for breast enhancement. The oil of these seeds can also be used directly on the breasts to improve firmness.

*Brussel sprouts* - are believed to regenerate and enhance breasts.

*Broccoli, cauliflower, peanut butter, and nuts* - are said to improve overall breast health.

## What to Avoid

Caffeine beverages such as coffee, tea, or soft drinks are believed to nullify the action of estrogen in the body. Therefore, it is recommended that caffeine be avoided.

# ROMANIA

Over the years, there has been a growing focus on women's health and beauty in Romania with nutrition and exercise playing a big part in this. Women generally desire thin yet fit bodies but as Romania is becoming more influenced by western ideas of the female body and femininity, that desire is changing.

In Brasov, in 1997, a Venus Beauty Program was conducted which was attended by over 50 women. The program demonstrated that by using perfectly natural methods, one's breasts could be radically transformed for the better in just three months.

After the program, it was concluded that the increases in breast size were obtained by applying the following methods:

**Nutrition**

Adopt a lacto-vegetarian diet, eating many fresh fruits and vegetables. Eat foods that promote breast growth like the following:

Black olives

Virgin olive oil

Soya, especially soya seeds

Wheat germ and wheat germ oil

Leaves, flowers and seeds of dill

Celery leaves

Walnut kernels

Roasted peanuts

Roasted sunflower seeds

As part of the program, it was recommended that these foods be eaten in large quantities for a minimum of 6 months.

## Herbal Blend

The following is a blend of herbs that is said to bring great results for breast enhancement.

Ingredients:

Dill seeds

Licorice root

Basil blossoms

Instructions:

1. With an electric coffee grinder, grind the ingredients into a powder.

2. Take 1 teaspoon of this mixture 3 times daily before meals. The mixture is to be put under the tongue for

fifteen minutes then swallowed with water.

## Breast Massage

Another method practiced by some Romanian women for breast enhancement is massage, which can be done with oils like wheat germ oil and dill. Massage techniques generally involve light moves back and forth on the breasts. These techniques have proven to be very effective in terms of firmness and breast lift when put into practice daily.

## Vacuum Therapy

Vacuum therapy is a deep massage that is performed by a special suction device. The cups used to create the suction stimulate milk ducts and thus increases blood pressure in the capillaries of the breasts, strengthening and toning the connective tissue.

## Breast Enhancing Meditation

One should not be fooled by appearances or the simplicity of this meditation. It is said to really do the trick if practiced every day. The meditation should be done immediately upon waking and in the evening, at least an hour before bedtime. Do not do this meditation too late or it is said to disrupt your sleep and you'll have a hard time trying to sleep.

Instructions:

Step 1.

Wash your face and hands and dress in something light – it's advisable to do this naked in the house but not necessary.

Step 2.

Close your eyes and silently count from 1 to 100 and then from 100 to 1.

Step 3.

Take in your hand two oranges or grapefruits or something similar - it is important that the size of the thing you hold in your hand to be similar to the breasts that you want.

Step 4.

Focus on the two oranges that you are holding in your hands. From time to time, slightly tighten the oranges in your hands and let them go as if you were squeezing your breasts.

Step 5.

Repeat mentally, "My chest is as big and strong as this orange (or whatever fruit you are using)."

Meditation should last between 10-15 minutes.

Tip - While doing this meditation, the effect is said to be greater if when you squeeze the oranges in your hands, think about a man you want and imagine he is squeezing your breasts. They say that the effects will be visible in about 2-3 months, no medication needed.

# RUSSIA

Since ancient times, Russian women aimed to look attractive and desired by men. The size of a female's breasts has always been an important factor and it still remains so today. Results of various polls and research show that Russian women have the largest average breast size of any country. For Russian men, the size and a shape of a woman's breasts are said to be an important factor and probably for this reason, Russian girls use various methods to make the breasts bigger.

So what are the most widespread techniques used to increase breast in Russia?

## Cabbage

Since ancient times, women who desired their breast to be bigger ate the following products: chicken, fish, dairy and fermented milk products, green apples, wine, and beer. However, the most ancient and perhaps the most popular product to increase the bust was cabbage. Mothers used this method and passed it down to their daughters. It should be noted that consumption of cabbage is said to be extremely effective when one is a teenager. As one ages, the efficiency decreases.

## Black Tea

Impressive effects are said to be achieved with the regular consumption of black tea with milk or tea from fresh strawberry leaves with milk. The tea stimulates an increase in a breast size according to many girls' opinions. A mix of walnuts with honey is sometimes added as a snack with the tea. This snack is easily prepared by just adding honey to walnuts.

## Bread Crusts

According to Russian women another way to increase a bust, , that is used everywhere in villages is to eat bread crusts. The myth states that after a half a year of eating bread crusts, it is possible to see quite good results with breast enlargement.

## Beer

Beer is another ancient folk remedy used to increase bust size. However, one should not buy all reserves of beer in the shop. It is said that not only does one experience an increase in breast size but also an increase in weight and alcoholism.

## Herbal Tinctures

Broths made from herbs are said to be beneficial for breast enhancement. For example, the following recipe has been passed down by mothers:

Take 1 tablespoon of hop cones and fill them with 1 glass of water.

Place on a water bath for 15 minutes, and then cool.

Take 2-3 tablespoons of this tincture 3 times a day.

The results are said to be amazing. Another effective tincture can be prepared from grains of rye, barley, millet, and corn. One should divide the mix into equal parts and add a lot of water. It is recommended that this mix be taken 3 times a day before meals.

## Cambrian Blue Clay (Russian Blue Clay) Mask

Cambrian Blue Clay or Russian Blue Clay is mineral rich and is said to increase blood circulation as well as stimulate collagen and cell growth. Applying the blue clay on the breasts overnight is said to be extremely effective at enhancing the breasts. The clay is also said to help tighten the breasts considerably and make the skin more elastic.

# SWEDEN

As one of the countries that is known for being open with a strong liberal democratic background, Swedish society is liberal about women and revealing tops that show off their breasts. In the summer months, it is not uncommon to see women wearing bikinis and sunbathing in a public park. There are also a number of beaches in the country that allow topless sunbathing and swimming.

In 2007, a network of women launched a campaign in Sweden for the right to bathe topless in the country's swimming pools. The movement was started when feminists heard about an incident involving two women in Uppsala. The two women were called ashore by a lifeguard when he saw them swimming topless. The movement called "Bara Bröst" (Just Breasts) called for the desexualization of women's breasts in society.

**Swedes Among the Biggest**

A worldwide survey in 2012 showed that Sweden is among the top countries whose women have the biggest breasts. The Scandinavians have one of the biggest cup sizes in the world with D as the average cup size. Russian women ranked number one.

## A Source of Magic

In the 18th century, young mothers were told to protect their breasts against the evil eye. It was the belief of the Scandinavian people that breast milk was a potent ingredient for magic and even witchcraft.

## Baby Oil and Cold Water

As a Nordic country, Sweden faces tough winters and the cold treatment does not end there. Some girls swear by massaging baby oil on their breasts and then rinsing it off with ice cold water. This method can efficiently be done while taking a shower and massaging one's breasts for three minutes. Rumor has it that the effects can be seen after just three days.

## Swedish Massage

Stimulating the breast tissue is one way of making them bigger, according to some Swedish ladies. With this 30-minute routine, all you have to do is put your right hand on your left breast and massage for 15 minutes. Repeat with the left hand and the right breast for another 15 minutes.

## Exercise

Swedes are known to be really health conscious, especially those who live in the city. A lot of women in Stockholm focus on their upper bodies during their gym sessions. Not only do these workouts make great arms but they also help make breasts look more firm and round.

# CHAPTER 3

# AFRICA

# GHANA

In some parts of Africa, certain rituals are conducted when an adolescent girl reaches puberty. These rituals are performed as a means of ushering the adolescent into womanhood. In Ghana, these acts are called Puberty Rites. Among the *Krobo* ethnic group this ritual is described as *Dipo* and among the Ashanti's it is known as *Bragoro*. It is during these rituals that young women are taught the secrets surrounding the achievement and maintenance of well-defined breasts and buttocks so that they can attract prospective husbands.

## Brief History Surrounding the Rites

In collaboration with some female opinion leaders and under the supervision of the queen mother of the town or village, young women who have had their first menstruation are secluded from the community for a period between two to three weeks during which they are taught the secrets of womanhood. During this period of seclusion, the girls are given lessons in sex education and birth control. They are also taught how to relate to men properly so they can maintain a good marriage and their dignity in society.

After the period of seclusion, a Durbar is held which is attended by the chief and almost everybody in the community. The newly initiated women are dressed scantily with very beautiful African beads and cosmetics accentuating their curves. Young men of marriageable age feast their eyes on the young women to select their prospective wives. On this occasion, the breasts are left bare for the young men to admire. The girls with the most beautiful, voluptuous breasts generally get selected first and are even contested for.

## The Secret to Naturally Larger Breasts

During the period of seclusion, the girls have their breasts smeared with special oils and ointments that will soften and enlarge the breasts to make them attractive to prospective husbands. The ingredients in the oil are purported to be blessed by the gods. They are also bathed with special medicinal plants, including leaves and barks from the Neem and Baobab trees, which according to traditions have spiritual healing powers. It is believed that these plants aid in the enhancement of their breasts and the whole body in general. The girls are taught how to routinely massage their breasts to give them that fullness and firmness to attract their husbands and, of course, they are also taught how to please their husbands in bed.

# NIGERIA

In Nigeria, there are tips and secrets from the days of old which help with breast enhancement. These methods were recommended to young brides largely from the southeastern parts of Nigeria such as Calabar, Akwa ibom, Abia, as well as the western parts like Oyo, Ogun, and a host of other geographical places therein.

Historical accounts state that most of these ladies were being prepared to be betrothed to their husbands. Many of these tips are still being used in these parts of Nigeria today. There are others that, in their haste, become impatient and neglect these age long secrets or tips because they would rather seek a very quick procedure that can be noticeable in hours rather than go through the slow process of natural breast enhancement.

These breast enhancement activities can take days, weeks, or even months before any results are seen. Those who have gone through these natural procedures claim that they are very effective and are better and safer than surgical procedures. Here are examples of Nigeria's age long secrets on breasts enhancement that are still being practiced today.

**Pawpaw Leaf**

The Pawpaw or Carica Papaya is a fruit that grows in South

America as well as in Africa. The papaya is a large, tree-like plant, with a single stem that grows from 5 to 10 m (16 to 33 ft.) tall with spirally arranged leaves found at the top of the trunk. This fruit is believed to cure a number of ailments including digestive disorders and intestinal parasites. In Nigeria, the elder women make it quite mandatory for any young maiden whose breasts are small and as a result aren't well rounded or appealing, to squeeze juice from a papaya leaf on to the nipples every morning for the breasts to become fuller and bigger.

## Pap

Pap is a very light, pasty meal made from maize. It is prepared and eaten in Nigeria and other African countries. Pap is made by soaking maize in water for a few days so that fermentation may take place. After about three days, the softened maize is then blended into a fine paste. It is then sieved so that the shafts may be separated from the meal. After all this has been done, it can then be prepared with hot water. Elder women claim that this can be a great breast enhancer. It is highly recommended that pap be eaten religiously, especially in the mornings, for one to get bigger breasts.

## Breast Massage

This is one secret that the elder women have held dearly and passed down for ages. It is said to be a time tested tip that has helped an avalanche of women and continues to be of immense benefit. Nigerian women believe that when the breasts are massaged for a long time with Shea butter, which is called *Ori* or *Okuma* in the Nigerian local languages, the breasts suddenly become noticeably fuller and bigger.

## Sucking Method

A long kept secret for breast enhancement is the sucking method. The myth advises that a woman who has small breasts to have them sucked by a man. This could either be her husband or an elder woman who is said to always be on standby. It is rumored to work wonders. Supposedly there are many who have undergone this process and have experienced good results.

# CAMEROON – A REVERSE CASE

While many in the western world spend thousands of dollars to be able to increase the size of their breasts, many countries in Africa do the contrary. A good example is Cameroon.

In Cameroon, some villages carry out a barbaric practice to stop the growth of breasts in young teenage girls. This practice is generally referred to as ''Breast Ironing''.

**What is "Breast Ironing"?**

Breast ironing is a very painful practice that involves massaging or pressing the breasts of young teenager with objects such as a heated wooden pestle, grinding stones, bananas, coconut shells, and spatulas. The aim is to retard the growth of the teen's breasts. Parents or close relations of the victims either convince the girls or force them to undergo this practice. When interviewed or questioned, parents who allow their children to undergo such practices give various reasons to justify their actions.

**Why Do Some Parents Practice "Breast Ironing"?**

According to parents who carry out this barbaric practice, their aim is to prevent sexual behavior in young teenage girls, prevent sexual harassment from men, and prevent them from rape and pre-teenage sex. Their end objective is to prevent unwanted pregnancies in teenage girls so the girls can complete their education successfully.

Contrary to the beliefs for this practice, sexual activities have not been curbed in teenage girls and hence have not prevented unplanned pregnancies. Rather, it has brought many negative effects on the girls that undergo this practice. Some victims complain of the inability as nursing mothers to produce breast milk, some turn out to have very large breasts, other develop breast cancer, which according to them, is caused by this practice. Other results include cysts and lesions on the breasts. Above all else, the practice is very brutal and painful and can lead to the destruction of delicate breast tissue.

# CHAPTER 4

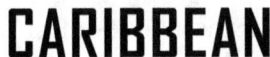

# CARIBBEAN

# JAMAICA

In Jamaican culture, men love curvy women. If your figure is puny, they are of the opinion that you look poor or are not taken care of. Jamaican women have a few myths about enhancing their breasts. The following traditional myths are those in which some Jamaicans believe. However, none of them are proven to be true.

### "I must, I must, I must increase my bust!"

One myth common in Jamaica amongst young preadolescence girls is to cross their arms above chest and use each hand to squeeze their biceps. While doing this they repeat "I must, I must increase my bust...I must, I must increase my bust." This practice is said to be done every day until an increase in breast size is seen for the believer.

### Fowl Pills

Fowl pills or chicken pills are used by many Jamaican women to not only increase bust size but also to increase the size of their backside and hips. Fowl pills are hormonal supplements that are given to chickens to increase their size and are not meant for human consumption. These pills can actually be very dangerous to humans as they can contain arsenic. Over time, the arsenic can build up and kill the person taking it.

## One Bubby Susan

Located in the Jamaican village of Woodside is a *Taíno* petroglyph (rock carving) of One Bubby Susan. Recorded in 1820, it is one of Jamaica's oldest known rock art sites, also known as Dryland. The petroglyph is called "One Bubby Susan" because she has only one breast. This is derived from the lore of Long or Lang Bubby Susan which legend says had breasts that touched the ground and when attacked, she would throw her breasts over her shoulder. Some women believe touching the rock carving will enhance their breasts.

## Herbs and Limes

Women in Jamaica belief that if they use creams made of different herbs their breasts will grow. Young teenagers also rub young limes on their chest as this is said to enhance the size of their breasts.

# ST. LUCIA

St. Lucia is a Caribbean island with approximately 170,000 people. It is one of the most beautiful islands and thus dubbed the 'Helen of the West'. As a result of the French and British conflicts, the people of St. Lucia speak two languages, English and Creole.

St. Lucia, like most of the Caribbean islands, has a very mixed heritage. It was first inhabited by the *Arawaks,* then the *Caribs,* and much later by the Europeans. The Europeans brought in the Africans and later Indians as indentured servants. While the island is largely composed of persons from African descent, there is a great mix of the other races found in most persons and as a result there is a mix of cultures and their beliefs.

The largely African heritage meant that women had ample breasts and really did not need enhancers of any kind. As a young girl, it can be a double edged sword. On the one hand a young girl, 10 or 11 years of age, begins to look at her body and wonders when her breasts will grow, especially if another girl her age has matured. However, a matured young girl with breasts feels self-conscious and different. She may dislike this change because some elders in the community may refer to her as "femme", a creole term used to say this young lady is advanced in her sexuality as if she caused her breasts to grow.

Young men growing up in rural communities quickly grow accustomed to seeing mothers with their breasts exposed while breastfeeding babies. Thus, breasts may not be novel to them. So the St. Lucian culture does not celebrate big breasts, just the opposite. A culture where smaller breasts, mind you not "no breasts", is just about perfect. Breast enhancement in adults is not a part of the culture and is hardly done.

In the rural communities, the use of herbs and using natural means for everything is part of the way of life. Words of wisdom, culture, myths, and herbal remedies were passed on from generation to generation. Most illnesses were treated with herbal remedies and so are enhancements of any body part. Growing up as a young girl, if you were unfortunate enough to be late in blossoming, you may have been eager to learn how to make your breasts grow and been tempted to try at least one of the following ways:

**Crayfish**

Those that live in the country generally live pretty close to a river and make frequent trips there. Especially during the summer, in order to bathe, have fun, and basically hang out with friends and get away from parents.

One myth for breast enhancement was to catch tiny crayfish and rub them on both breasts. Do it gently, so as to not crush them, then drop the crayfish back into the river. The premise was that as the crayfish grew, so would your breasts.

## Calabash

The calabash tree bears round, hard, fruit-like calabashes. Long ago, the calabash, which has a hard shell, was cut in half and the non-edible pulp was removed. The shell was then dried in the sun and used as bowls and cups. The calabash is still used as such in many traditional Creole activities.

One tradition was to climb the calabash tree or use a low hanging branch to find a small calabash fresh out of the flower bud. One would rub their breasts with the newly formed fruit and as the fruit grew to its big round size (hopefully not too big), so would one's breasts.

## Saliva of a Newly Pregnant Cow

This myth was more commonly used by young boys who wanted to grow a bigger penis but this myth also applied to girls who had hopes of growing bigger breasts. It was mostly done by young girls who lived on a farm and were comfortable around female cows. The saliva or drool of a newly pregnant cow was collected and rubbed onto one's breasts with the premise that as the baby cow grew, so would your breasts.

Were these methods used by many young ladies and did they work? Now, older folks jokingly say that they remember trying at least one of these methods. The most tried method was rubbing crayfish on one's breasts. However, the one most believed to have worked is the calabash method. The belief is that the crayfish could easily be caught and die, hence your breasts would not grow any further while the calabash survival was a lot more assured, especially now that the use of it as utensils has greatly diminished.

# CHAPTER 5

❖

# SOUTH AMERICA

# ARGENTINA

The Argentinean society likes big breasts. National movies and magazines are covered with big breasted women. Miss Argentina of 1955, Isabel Sarli (aka "La Coca Sarli"), was maybe the first exponent of this "big breast girl" movement. She was a cultural icon and sex symbol in Argentina. Many more actresses since have been viewed as sex symbols like Moria Casan during the 70's and 80's.

With bigger breasts being part of the culture, some women in Argentina try to increase their breast size by the following methods:

**Eating Chicken**

Amongst teenagers, there is a rumor that eating chicken will make your breasts grow. This is because many chicken hatcheries use growth hormones so they can sell bigger chickens. Teens believe that eating chickens treated with hormones result in one's breasts growing. This myth is totally refuted by doctors but young girls still believe it.

## Sex

Some people in Argentina believe that the more sex one has, the bigger the breasts will become. If a woman is excited and a man is massaging her breasts, it is rumored that the breasts will grow within a few days.

## Ice

Like many European countries mentioned in this book, massaging the breasts with ice is believed to maintain firm and younger looking breasts. Simply get a piece of ice and rub it throughout the chest without touching the nipples.

## Massage

Massaging the breast is said to increase blood circulation to the breasts. Using any kind of cream or lotion works. Massage each breast in a circular motion from the center and out without touching the nipple.

## Breast Enhancement Patches

Breast enhancement patches and other breast enhancing supplements can be found in Argentina. The patches contain breast enlarging herbal extracts and are adhesive which allows them to be worn on the skin. The product in the patch is easily absorbed through the skin. The benefit of the patch, as believed by some, is that the breast enhancing products absorb directly into the bloodstream and bypass the liver.

# BRAZIL

Taking care of and maintaining one's body is common among Brazilian women. This is done by working out and getting beauty treatments often. The ideal body for a Brazilian woman is fit and toned with nice buttocks and medium-to-large breasts. Plastic surgery is common in Brazil but for those who cannot afford it or maybe are just curious, natural remedies are available that promise to increase the size of their breasts. Here are a few of the many superstitions and myths that can be found in Brazil for natural breast enlargement.

### Corn + Chicken + Patience

One superstition involves the use of three grains of corn, a chicken, and patience to perform the ritual for 13 weeks. For this myth to work, it is said that the woman needs to imagine her breasts growing while taking the first grain of corn and passing it three times around her nipple. The process should be repeated on the other breast. The women will need to do the same process with the second and third grain of corn. Lastly, she needs to give the three grain of corn to a rooster or a chicken to eat. The ritual must be repeated in the same process for thirteen Fridays in a row and she is to not tell anyone about what she is doing.

## Milk and Holy Water

Another superstition requires milk, water, holy water, and cotton. This ritual needs to be performed for 30 minutes every day for three consecutive days. First, the woman is required to mix 1/2 cup milk plus 1/2 cup water and 7 drops of holy water. Next, she is to wet two cotton balls into the mixture and place a cotton ball in each bra cup. Wait 15 minutes, then the women will need to throw the mixture and the cotton balls away. According to the superstition, this 15 minute ritual must be repeated twice a day for three consecutive days.

## Green Coconut Water

This myth involves green coconut water, an ice tray, a refrigerator, and one week of time. The woman needs to make ice cubes with the green coconut water. Before going to bed, she needs to get one of the ice cubes and rub it on her breasts in a circular motion, starting from the left breast and then moving to the right breast. This process must be repeated on each breast until the ice cube has melted to where it is difficult to hold. When the ice cube gets to this point, the woman needs to put it in her mouth and suck on it until it is gone. The myth states that the breasts must dry naturally. This ritual must be repeated daily for a week, beginning and ending on a Friday.

Breast Massage

There are also massage techniques in Brazil that promise to enhance the breasts, keep them lifted and prevent sagging. Massaging the breasts also helps in the release of a hormone known as prolactin, which assists in breast growth. It is recommended that one use rosehip oil or almond oil to facilitate the hand movements without causing friction. These oils also have nutrients that hydrate and tone the skin. Essential oils can be added as well.

One massage technique used by Brazilian women consists of holding one breast with one hand and proceeding to make circular movements for 15 minutes, then doing the same thing on the other breast for another 15 minutes. The woman must be careful not to tug on the skin as this is said to contribute to the disruption of the fibers that help support the breasts. The morning or before bedtime are said to be the best times of day to perform the massage. With patience and discipline, it is said that one should start seeing results in about 5 weeks.

Another technique for breast enhancement is done as if a woman were cradling a child. The hands should be crossed and on the outer sides of the opposite breasts. The hands should be brought together to squeeze the breasts together. It's recommended to do it once a day for ten minutes.

More Secrets and Myths

Chest muscle exercises also help to increase and strengthen the breast region. The muscles help to support the breasts. One way to do this is with the use weights. If there are no gym weights at home, bags of rice or sugar are said to provide the same effect, according to women in Brazil.

The breasts are a very sensitive part of the body. They may lose their elasticity easily which results in a loss of support. To avoid these problems, wearing the correct size bra is always recommended. Avoid wetting the breasts with very hot water when bathing and always use creams or lotions to keep the skin on the neck, décolleté, and breasts hydrated. The skin of the chest and the neck help to support the breasts.

Drinking lots of water assists in the renewal of cellular nutrients. Also, consuming protein is said to promote cell rejuvenation. It is recommended that one use a sports bra or supportive top whenever doing physical exercise such as walking, cycling, aerobics, dancing, or high impact activities which help to keep the breasts supported. It is believed that losing and gaining weight several times can be negative for the appearance of the breasts.

# CHILE

In Chile, the desire for different body types is generally based on class. The high class or rich women generally desire to be thin and tall with small breasts. While some middle class women desire to be tall and thin, many middle class and lower class women desire to have curves with big breasts and butts. Natural methods used to achieve their desires are:

**Eating Chicken**

Some Chilean women eat chicken every day, not necessarily because this is their favorite food but because it is rumored that these animals are injected with hormones which are believed to promote breast enlargement in humans.

**Soymilk**

Many women in Chile believe drinking a liter of soymilk daily is beneficial to breast growth. They believe that soy's high content of natural estrogen is supposed to help the breasts grow very quickly.

## Gain Weight

In Chile, some women try to achieve their dreams of beautiful breasts by gaining weight because they believe this will result in increased breast size. However, there are also women who believe weight gain is not the answer because they believe that the increased weight can actually make the breast sag and become less firm.

## Lemon and Tomato Juice

A myth in Chile states that drinking tomato juice with lemon will enlarge one's breasts. It is said that this concoction is given by some men to their women who they desire to have larger breasts. This myth is said to have been passed down through the generations in Chile.

## Grape Juice

Some women in Chile believe that if one massages their breasts with grape juice, their breasts will grow considerably.

## Breast Massage

It is believed by many that squeezing one's breasts for a few minutes every day will result in enlarged breasts. It is a habit that is said to have been practiced by many women in Chile and is still practiced today.

# MEXICO

Even though we are in the 21st century, in most regions of the country, it is still taboo to speak about breast size. This is something one should not speak about in an everyday conversation with friends, especially if you do not live in a capital city. Information about sexuality is still restricted and not spoken about publicly in marginal areas of the country. People of society's high classes are more likely to speak about this and other sexual topics more openly.

**Fennel Seed Tea**

Women in Mexico believe that fennel seed tea helps increase breast size. This tea is also said to help new mothers increase their milk supply. A simple recipe for the tea is to boil 1/2 liter of water and 1 spoon of fennel seed. Let seep for 10 minutes then drink 3 times a week for breast enhancement.

**Oatmeal Atole**

Atole is a Mexican comfort food that is generally made of oats, water, milk or both, and cinnamon. It is thinner than traditional oatmeal and is usually served as a beverage. Some women in Mexico believe that one should drink 1 to 2 cups of atole, three times a week to increase breast size. Atole is also used by many new mothers in Mexico to help increase milk supply. Eating too much can result in weight gain which might be the reason why some women notice an increase in breast size from eating too much atole.

## More Foods for Breast Enhancement

Soya products are known for their breast enhancing properties among women in Mexico. Grandmothers recommend eating the following products, in any of its forms: yogurt, milk, cheese or stewed, as a daily meal. Chickpeas and apples are also said to increase breast size. Apples can be eaten every day and the chickpeas should be eaten at least 2 times a week for optimal results.

## Breast Masks

There are a number of homemade breast masks that Mexican women believe assist with natural breast enhancement.

*Egg White Breast Mask*

Beat one egg white until stiff then massage onto breasts and let stand for about 30 minutes. Wash off with cold water. Do these three times a week for best results.

*Banana Puree Breast Mask*

Mash or puree one ripe banana (maybe 2, depending on the size). Apply the puree over your breast, avoiding the nipple area. Leave the puree on the breasts for 25 minutes then rinse off with cold water. Rumor has it that applying this breast mask twice a week will provide good results.

Share Your Secrets and Myths

Do you have a breast enhancement secret, myth, or legend from a country that is not listed or would you like to expand on one that is?

This book is an on-going project and any contributions to make this a robust resource of secrets and myths from around the world are welcomed.

Please email your secrets and myths to:
secrets@projectgoodies.com

# Books by Alexa Reyna

## Breast Massage and Acupressure
### for Improved Breast Health and Increased Fullness

For more information on natural breast enlargement, visit

www.growbreastsnaturally.com

www.ingramcontent.com/pod-product-compliance
Lightning Source LLC
Chambersburg PA
CBHW071158280526
45787CB00002B/542